A Tale of Two Jews
Nehemiah & Ezra

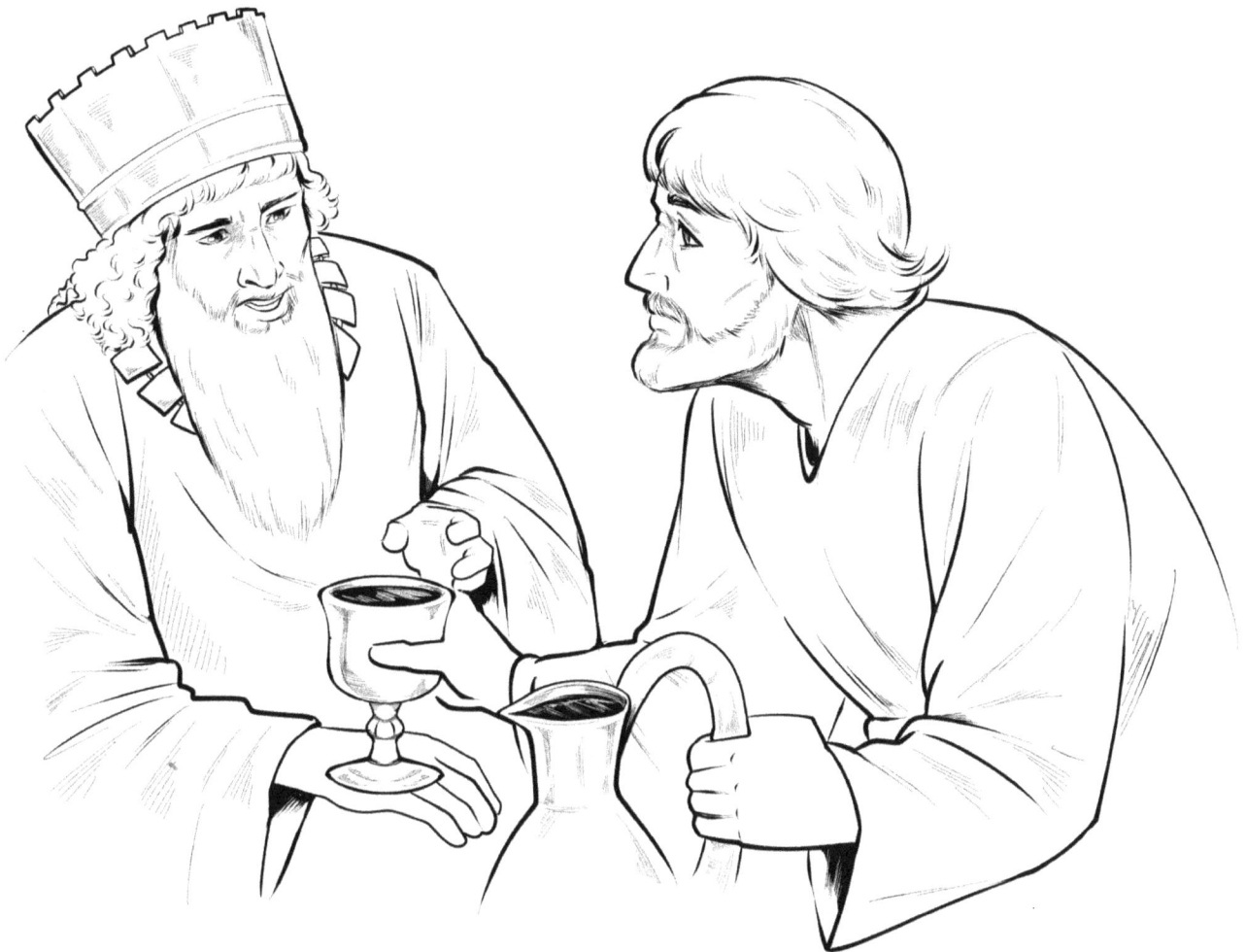

Illustrated Bible Story by Shirley A. Franklin

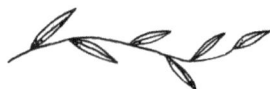

A Tale of Two Jews: Nehemiah & Ezra

Copyright 2024 © Shirley A. Franklin

Writezous Publishing
301 S. Heatherwilde Blvd, #51
Pflugerville, Tx 78660-9998

ISBN 978-0-9778520-3-1

This story is an adaptation from the books of Ezra and Nehemiah in The Holy Bible.

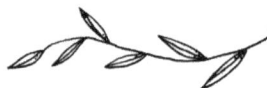

"The common laborers held a
TOOL
in one hand and
a spear in the
other.

Each of the
builders had a
SWORD
strapped to his
side as he
worked."

**Nehemiah
4:17**
(The Message)

Nehemiah used his strong, slender fingers to pull up the folds of his long, flowing robe to go into the palace's foyer to see who had come to visit him at King's Art's palace. It was a beautiful place with the best of everything. Nehemiah was the king's cupbearer, a man who tasted the king's drinks before giving them to the king. This was a job with the chance that he was sacrificing his life. For if the drink was poison, Nehemiah would die instead of the king. When you are a king, there could be people who might try to take your life by sending a poisoned bottle of wine disguised as a friendly gift.

Nehemiah was someone who the king trusted. As he hurried down the hall, with his triple striped sandals making shst tuss shst tuss shst sounds on the geometric tiles, he wondered who his visitor might be. Nehemiah only looked down once, beholding the tiles beneath his wide feet – they were made of triangles, squares and tilted squares of natural hues like beige, brown and camel. During this glance, he lifted his robe higher, revealing strong muscular legs and thick, squarish knees.

The heavy five foot wide and ten-foot-tall walnut-colored double doors of bars and wooden beams were opening, as two of the king's servants were allowing the visitors inside.

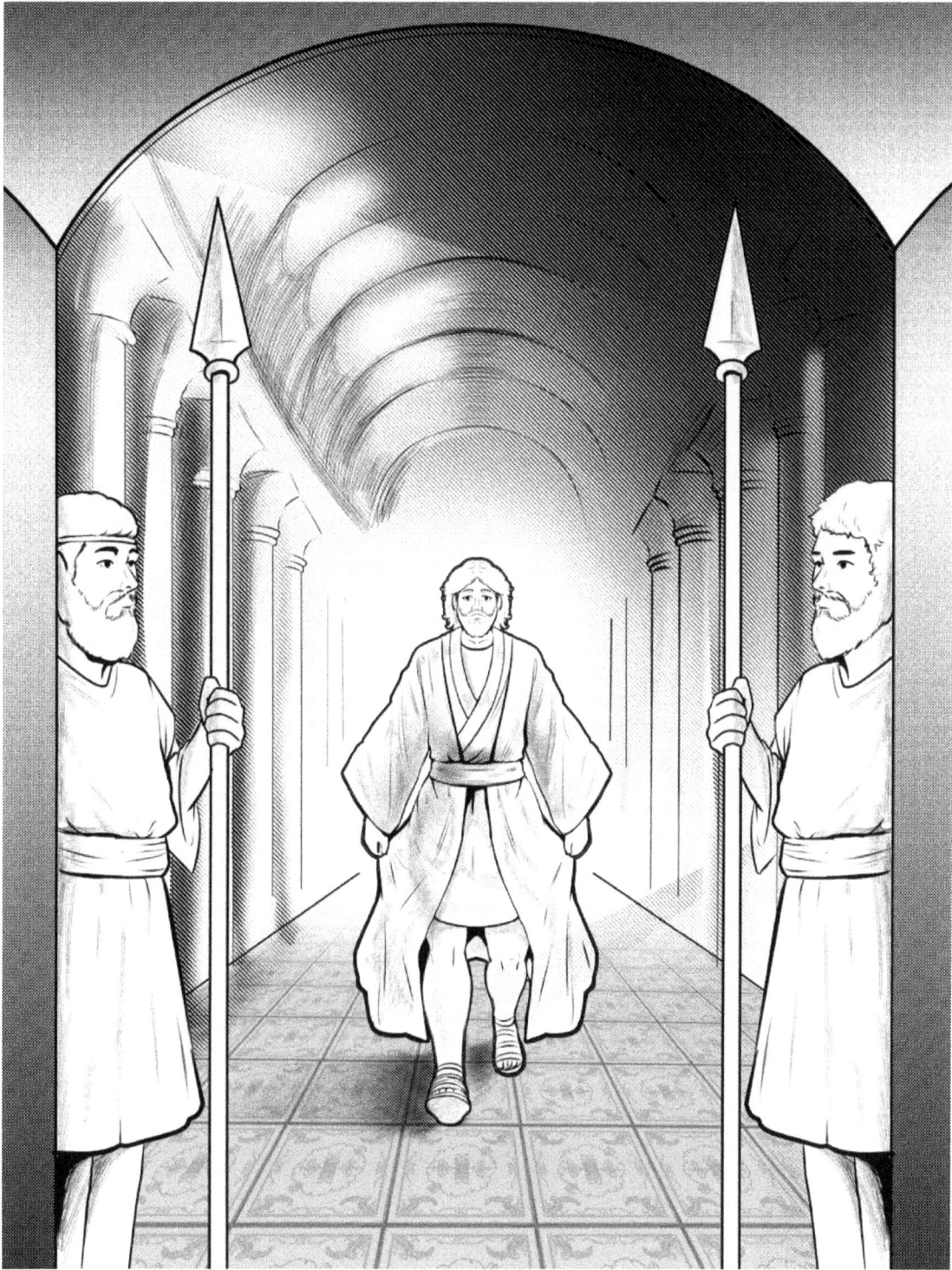

Dapples of sunlight splashed into the foyer from behind the men as they walked into the palace and sat near the entrance on carved wood framed cushioned velour seats which were backed with nail-heads every 2 inches creating puffy stuffed diamond shapes all across the back. The tall, slender man who was leaned back enjoying the comfort of the seats, leaned forward as Nehemiah broke into a grin. He recognized a Jewish brother from before the Babylonian captivity. He didn't know the men with him.

After they embraced and then sat together, Nehemiah asked about Jerusalem, the city where God dwells (Psalm 46:4) and those who had returned home there. The friend's shoulders slumped over before he answered. This heavily bearded friend looked him in the eyes and broke the news, "The people are in shame and the walls and gates are run-down and burned."

Nehemiah's shoulders slumped more and more as he listened. They talked about other matters, but Nehemiah's mind kept going back to the bad state of the sacred city and the Jews who he dearly loved. In his mind, he saw lots of rubble, cracked stones laying all across the ground just about everywhere one looked. He saw people in tattered clothes wandering around, killing time with no sense of direction.

He prayed about the sad news he'd just heard. He asked God to remember how He had taken care of His people in the past. He asked God to forgive them for ignoring His warnings and to give them another chance. He asked God to give him support from the king. Again, he could picture in his head what things looked like back home as he prayed.

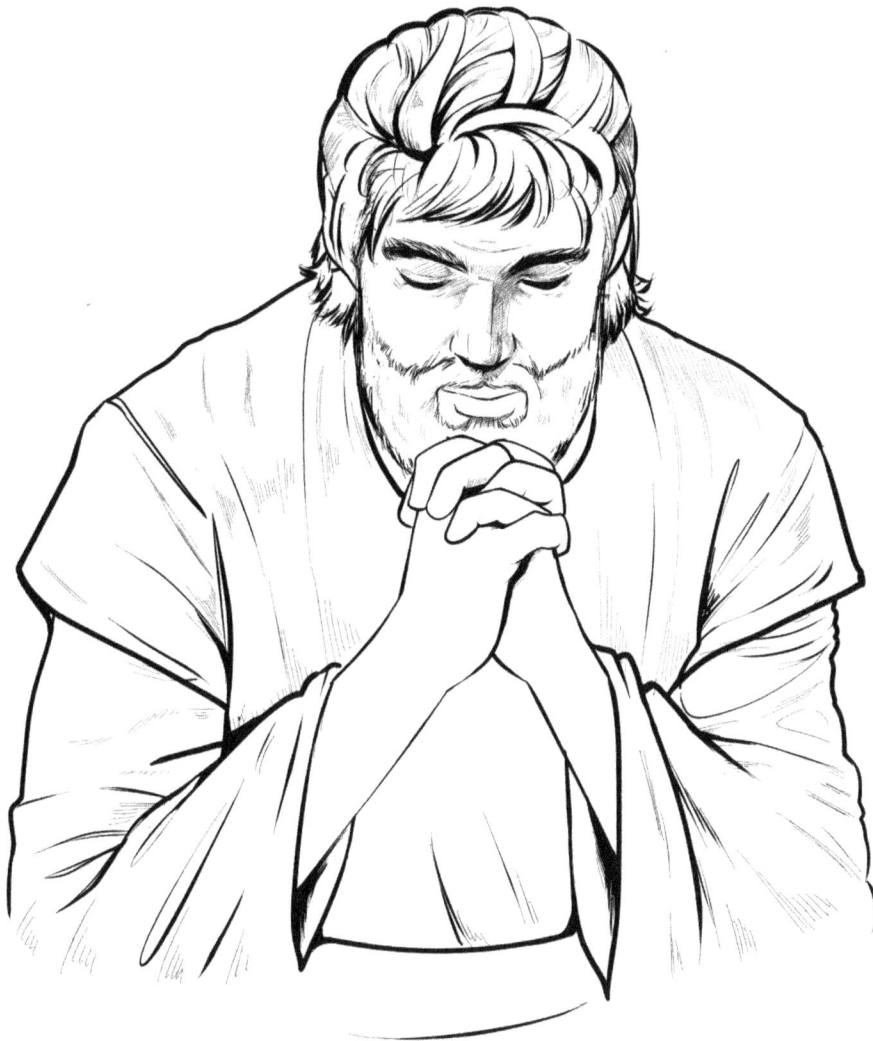

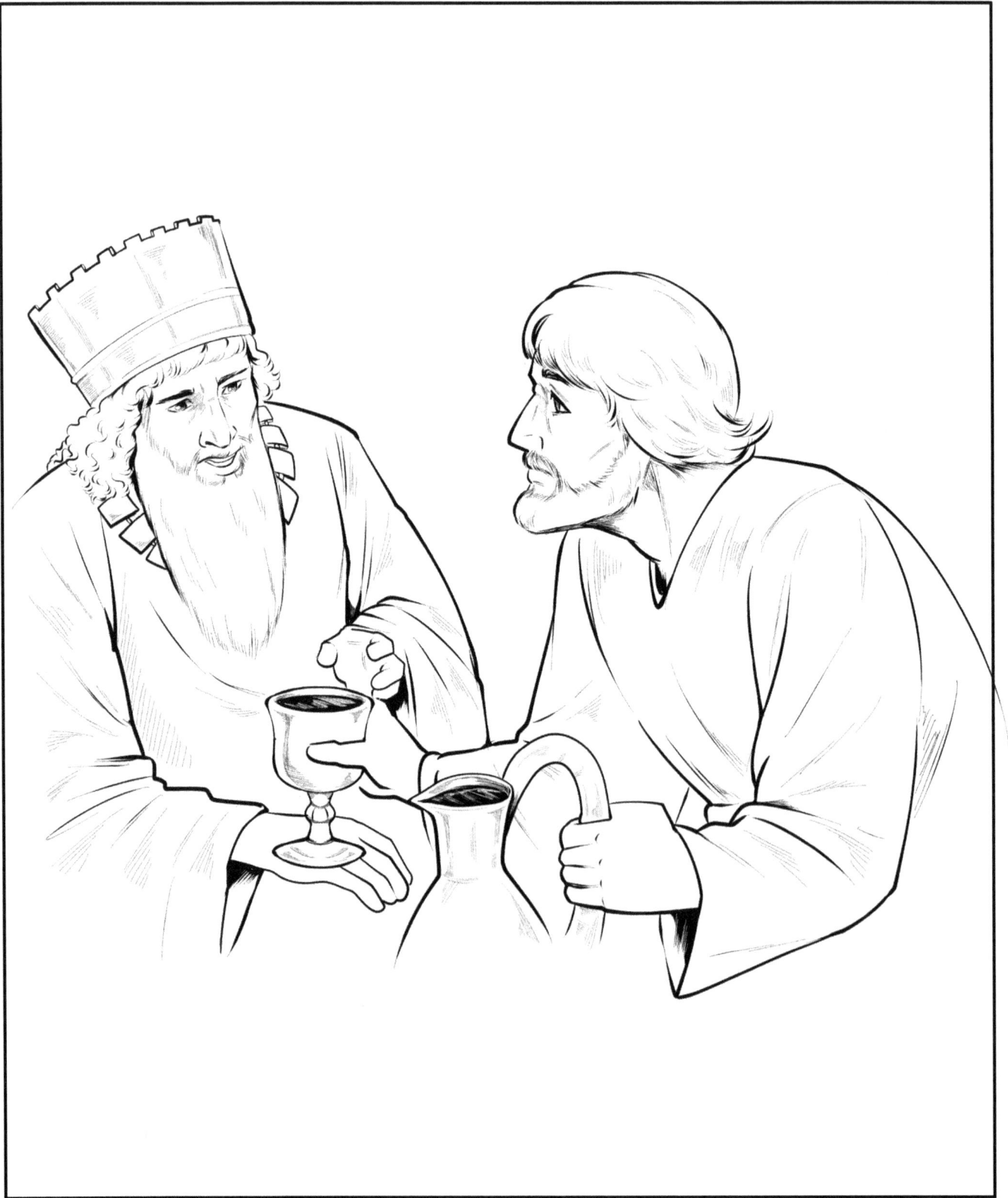

As he poured the king's sparkling dark purple drink later, he looked sad. This was something new, as he was normally happy and joyous.

"Why so sad?" The king asked.

"My beloved Jerusalem is in ruins. It breaks my heart. A friend who visited me earlier today told me that the Jews there are in a state of disgrace and the walls and gates are in ruins."

"What would you ask of the king?" Queried King Art. He shifted in his seat to look at his cupbearer.

"If I could go back home, I could lead the project to rebuild Jerusalem and help my fellow Jews," said Nehemiah, his almond-shaped honey brown eyes brimming with tears.

The king agreed to let Nehemiah leave, then wrote letters that gave him permission to make the trip and to get the timber wood that he needed for the project. The king used melted red wax from a long, tapered candle to create a puddle at the bottom of the letters. He then used a signet ring on his finger, which had a special design, his emblem and his initials on it to press into the wax. Anyone viewing the letters would believe that the letters came from the king, and that they were not fake. The king also sent special people to help Nehemiah.

Nehemiah arrived back home. Soon after arriving on his secret mission, he arose at night and traveled with a few men to take a look at the walls. Sure enough, the walls were in bad shape and the gates had been burned with fire. There was so much crumbled and blasted rubble, that at some points, they had to get off their stout, shiny black horses and walk.

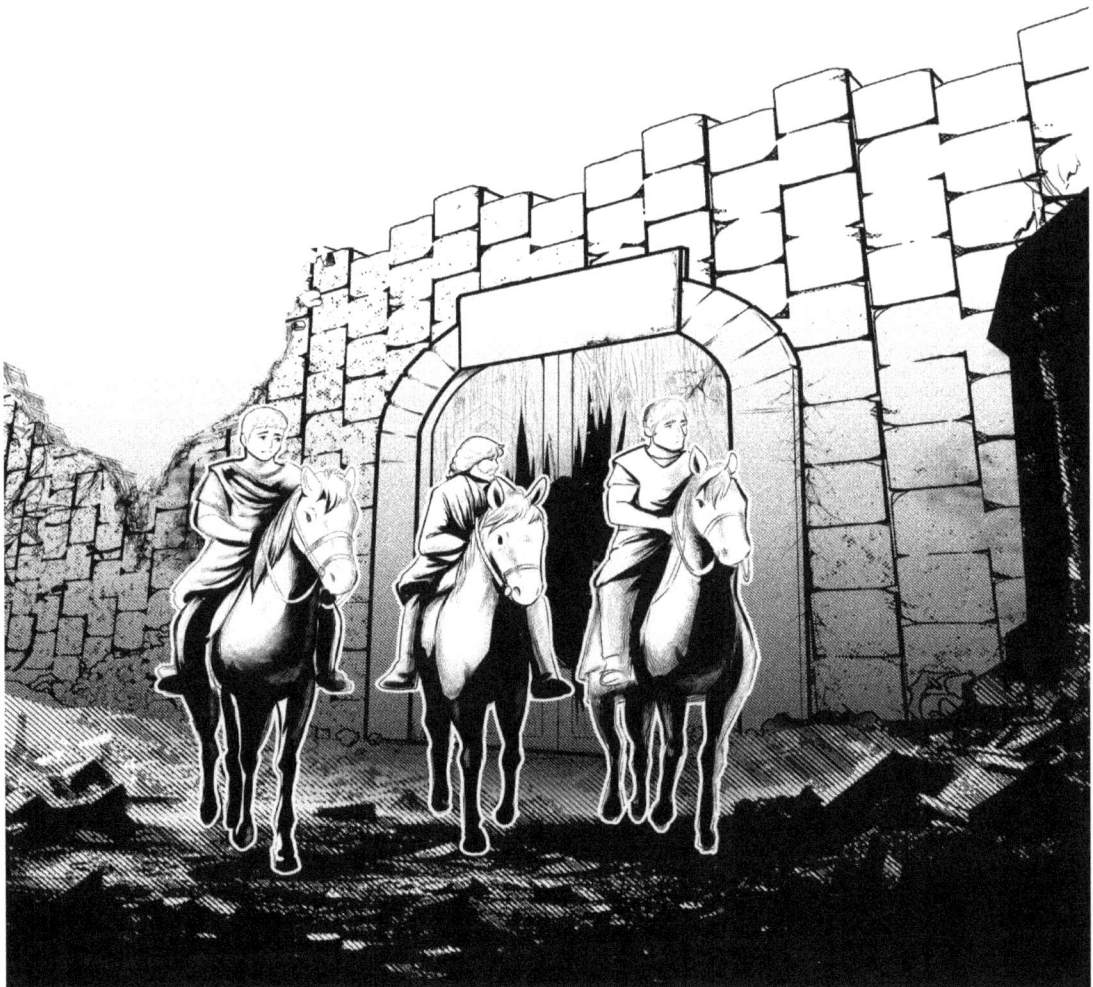

People who he reported to asked some questions and then agreed to go help with the rebuilding project. They were satisfied with the answers Nehemiah gave. He told them that God would give them success.

They said, "Let's start rebuilding."

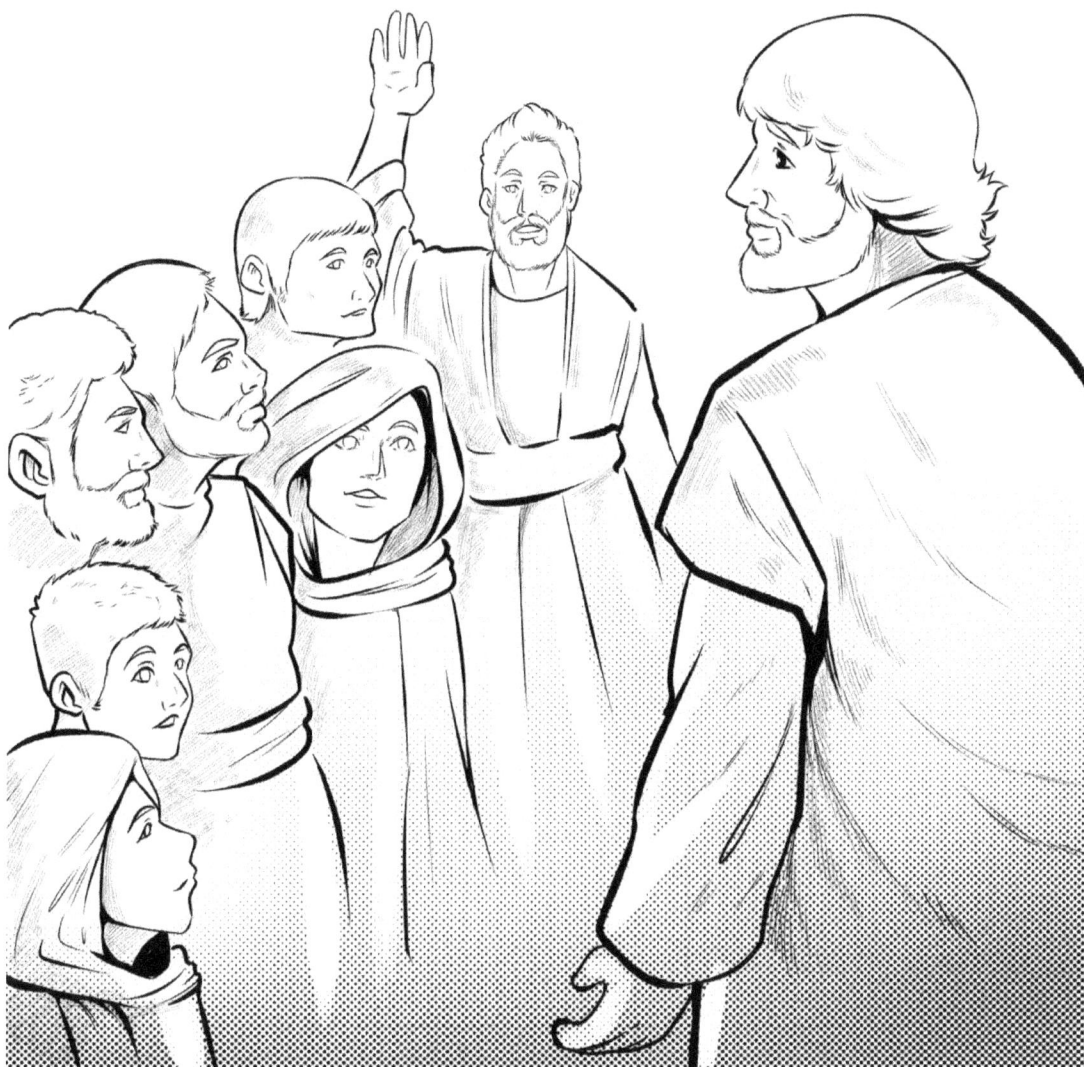

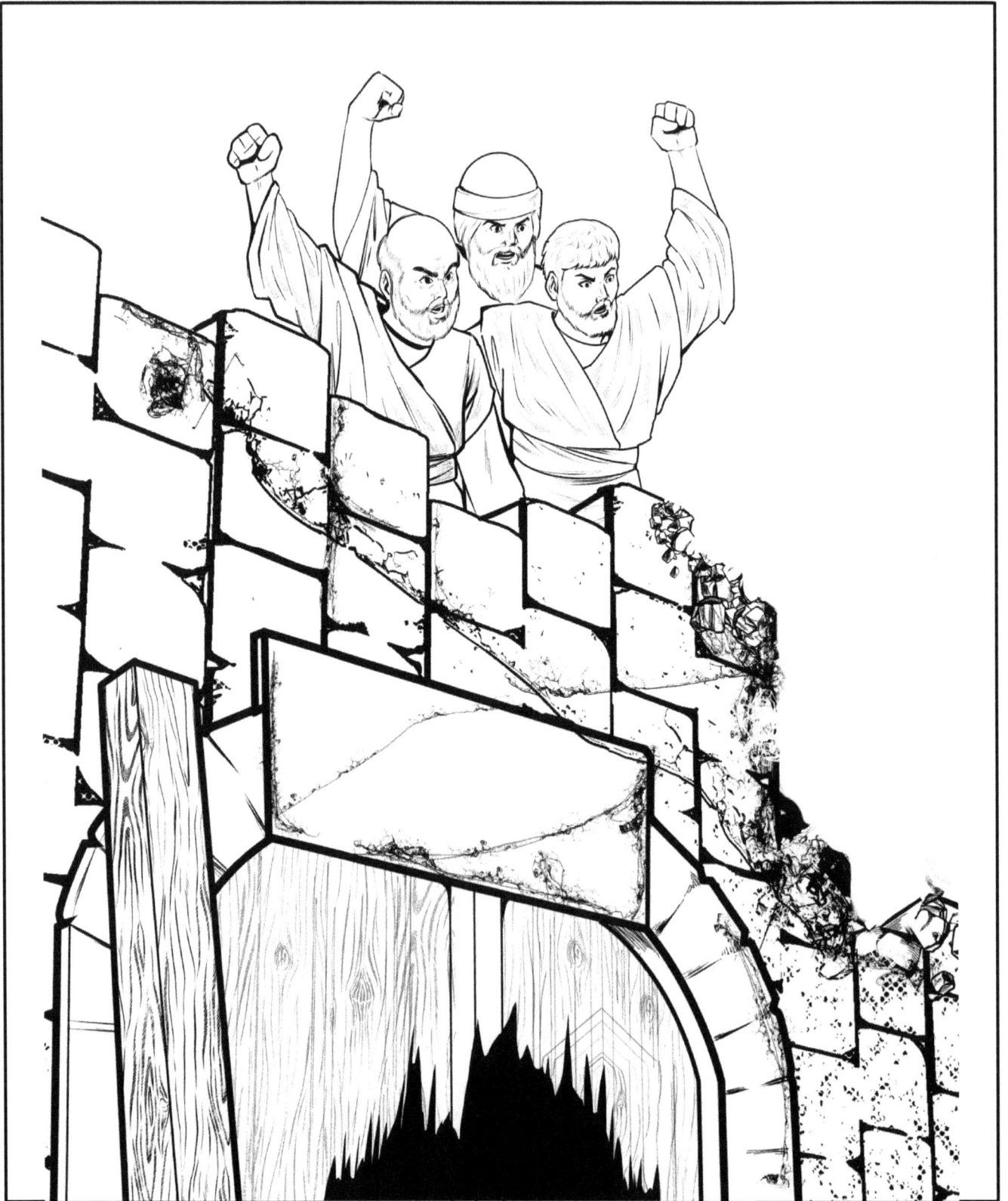

Three stubborn enemies did not want the rebuilding to take place. They found Nehemiah and asked him a question that had a hidden threat.

"Are you rebelling against the king?" They said.

"We are God's servants. You have nothing to do with Jerusalem," Nehemiah told them.

San, Toby, and Gersh showed their anger. Their eyes flashed and they furrowed their foreheads. One even raised his fist. These three got angrier and angrier as the rebuilding continued. They even tried all kinds of tricks, threats, wicked plans and plots to stop or distract the workers and Nehemiah. They pointed out that the area was full of burnt stones and mountains of rubble.

The builders let Nehemiah know that many people were trying to bother and attack them.

They told him, "Everywhere you turn, they attack us."

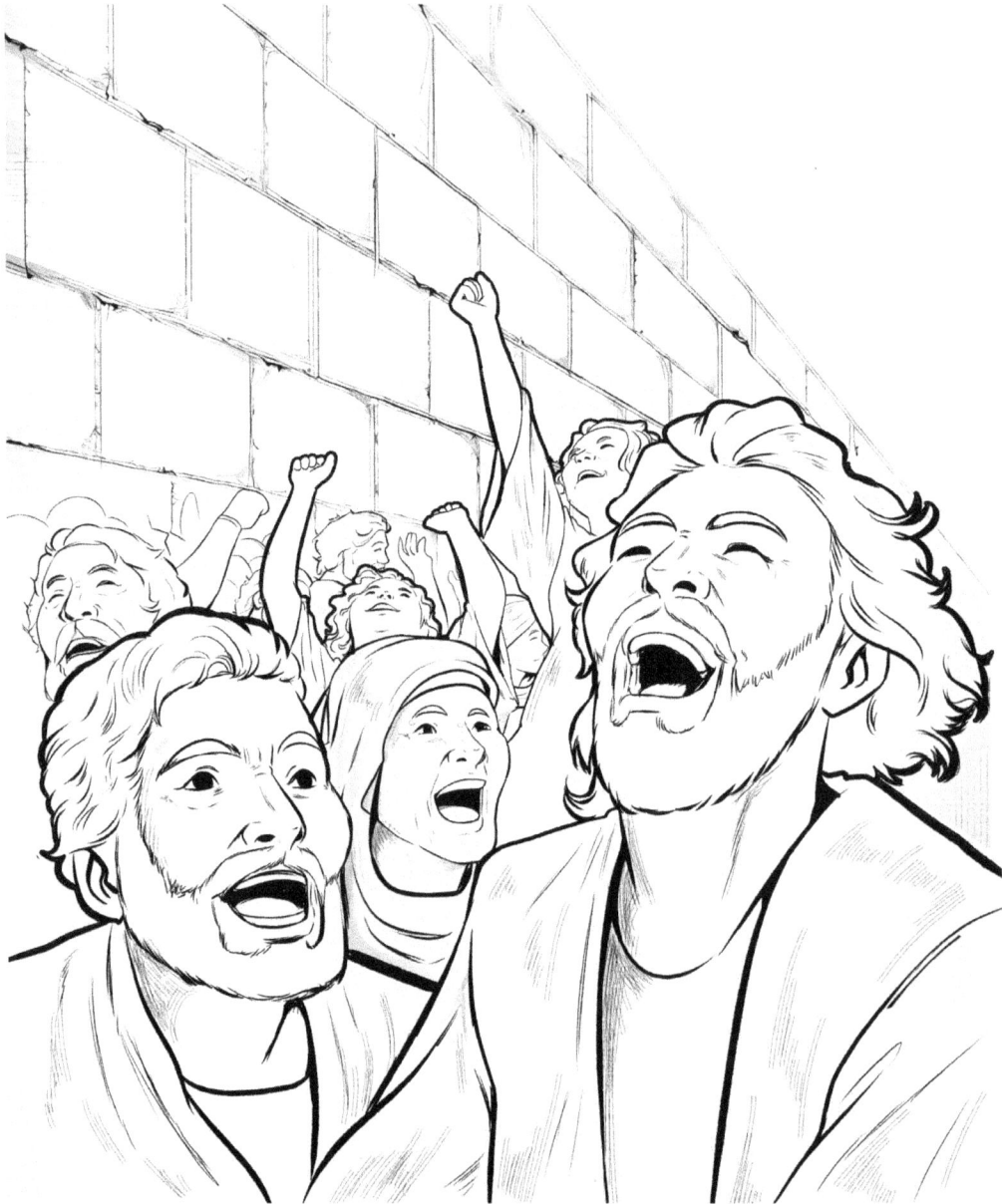

He gave people jobs guarding the walls by holding weapons in case they needed to fight. Some were in family groups, holding spears, swords and bows.

"Don't be afraid. Remember that you are doing this for your families," Nehemiah told them.

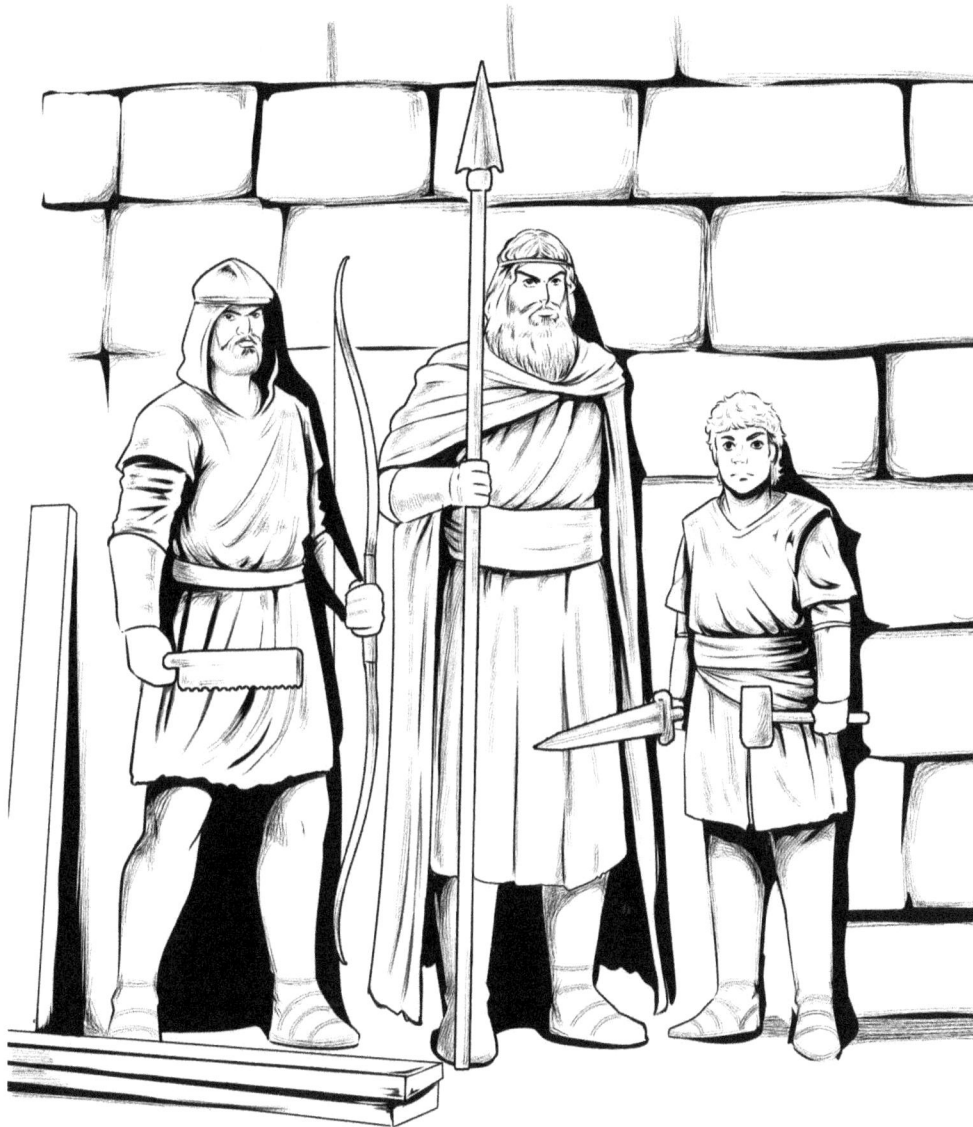

They continued their work, with some families, merchants temple servants, priests, rulers, Levites, perfumers and goldsmiths making repairs to walls, houses, and gates.

Others worked at building gates. Even daughters helped their fathers at sections assigned to their families by installing doors, gates and bars.

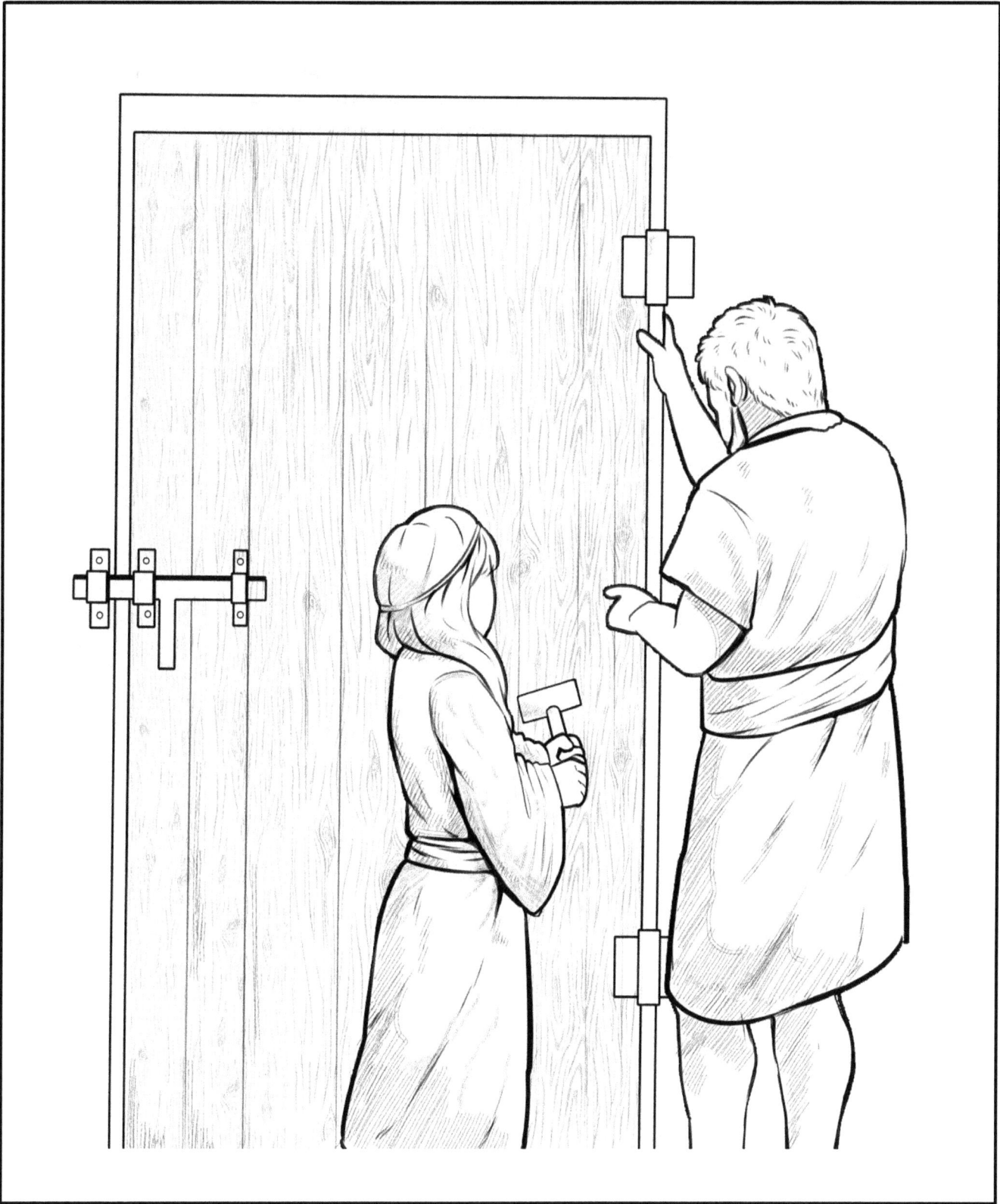

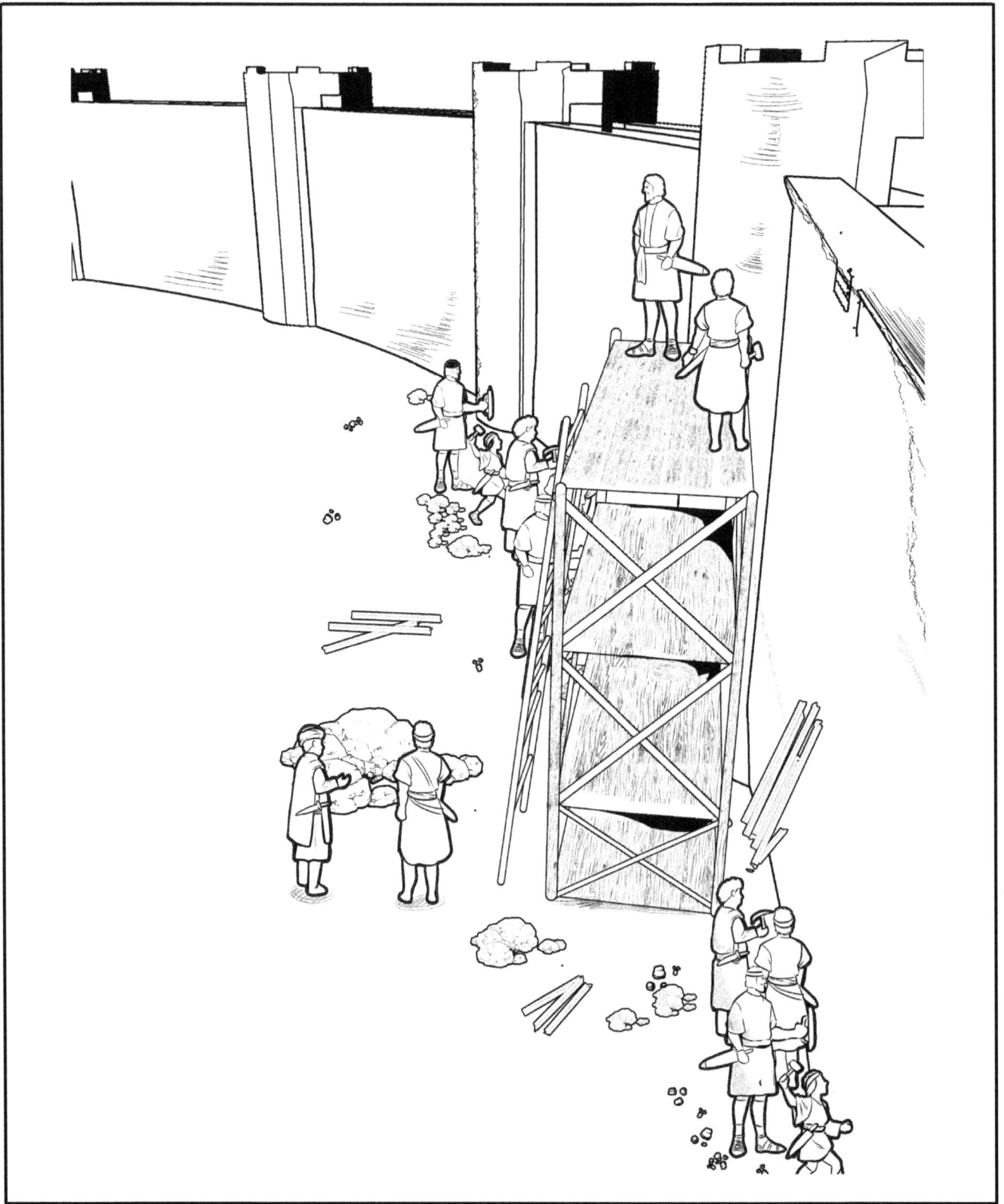

Workers and laborers worked on the walls with a tool in one hand and a fighting weapon in the other hand.

Nehemiah told the people that since they were all spread out and there was lots of work to do, he had a safety strategy. "Whenever you hear the trumpet sound, rally to us here. God will do the fighting." Nehemiah kept the trumpeter by his side.

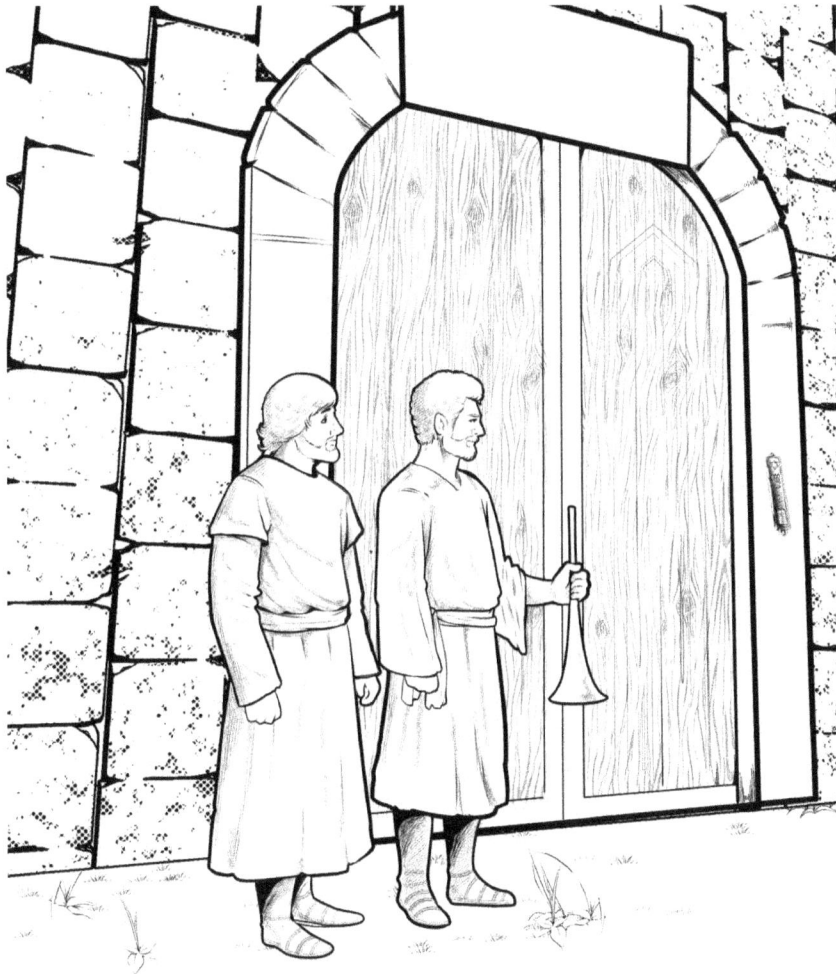

While building continued, Nehemiah assigned some men to stand guard and hold spears from the early part of the day until the stars visited the sky.

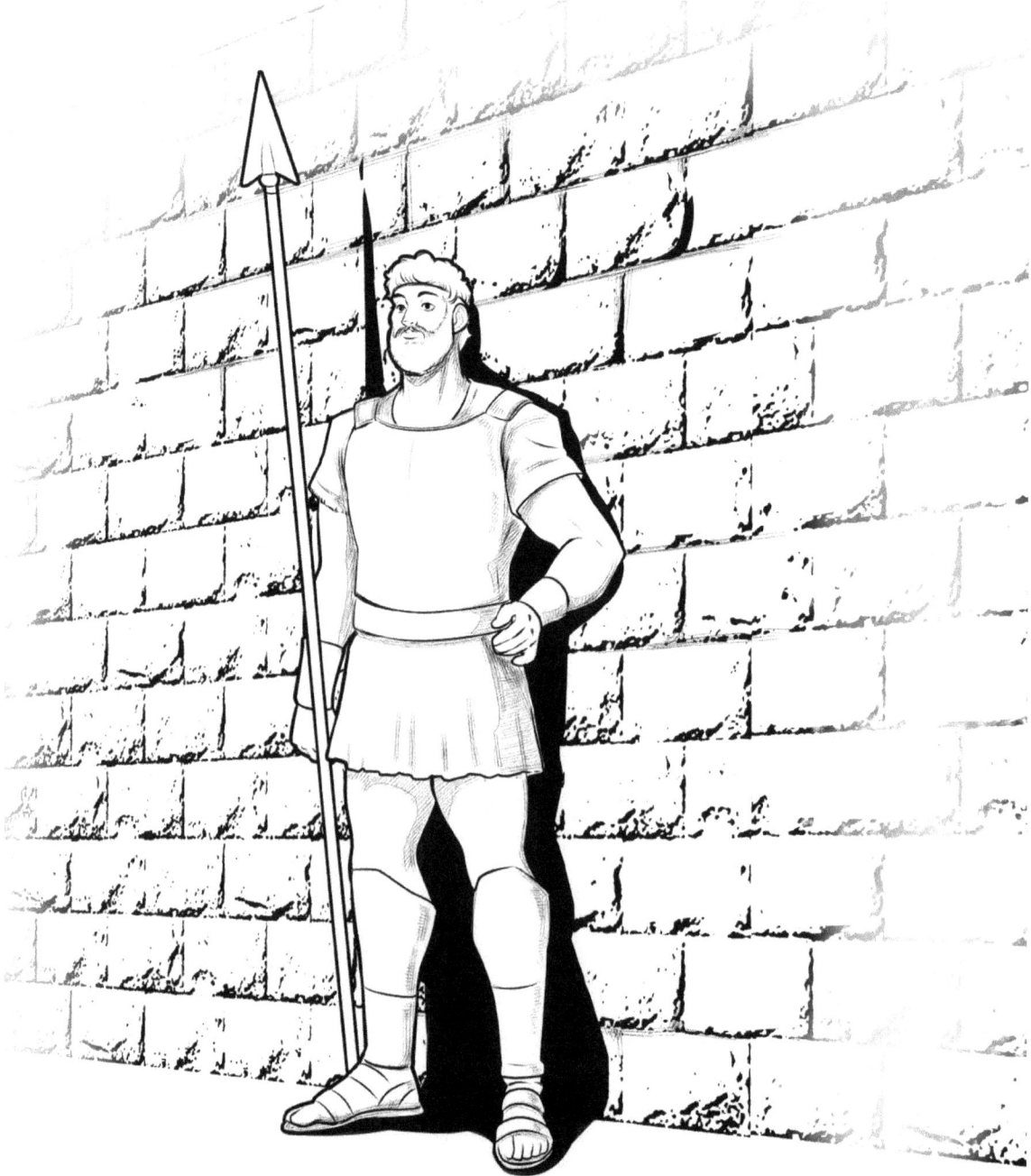

He even told them to take their weapons when going to nearby waterways to get water.

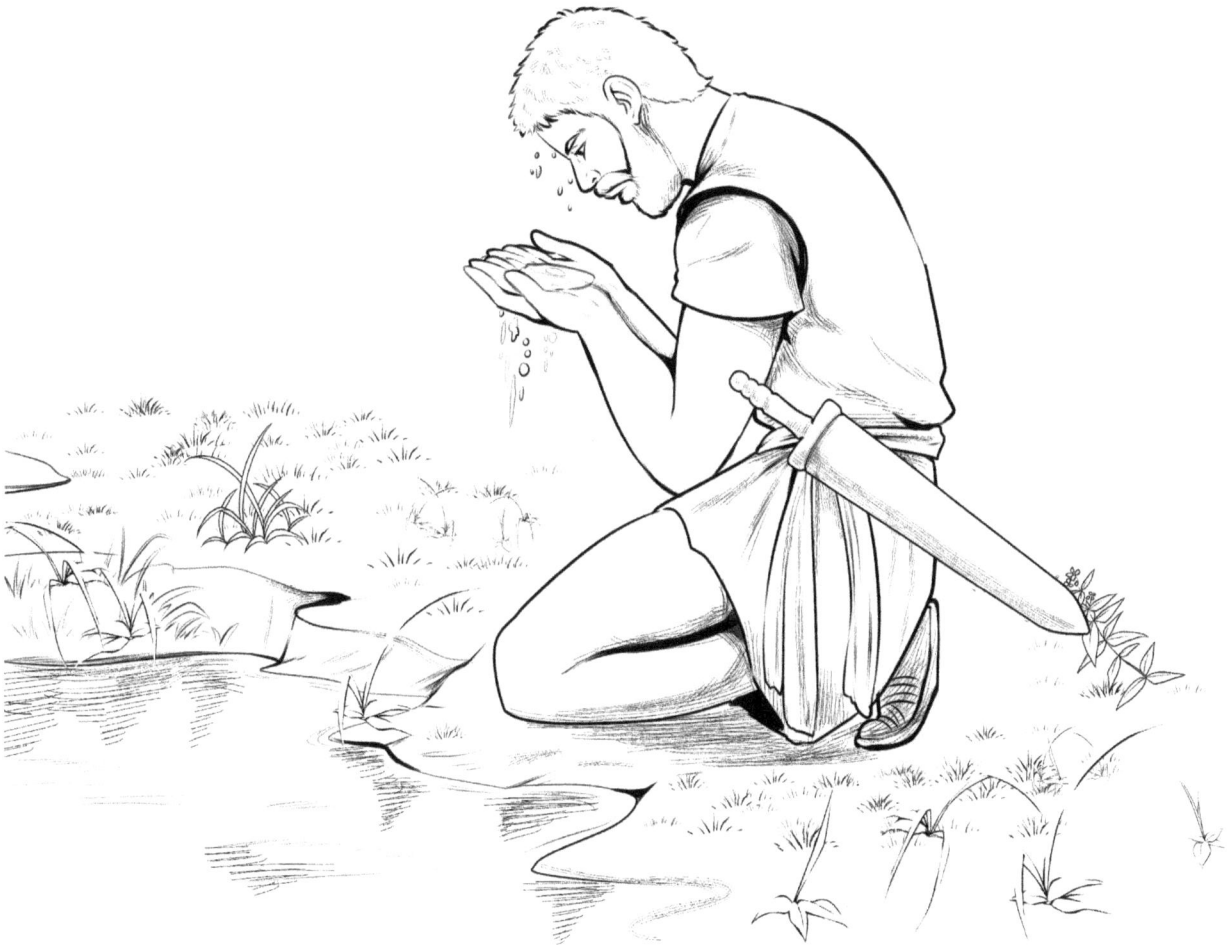

The troublesome trio tried to get Nehemiah to come down from the wall. He knew this would require that he stop rebuilding. He replied, "I'm doing a great work, and I can't come down." He then asked God for strength.

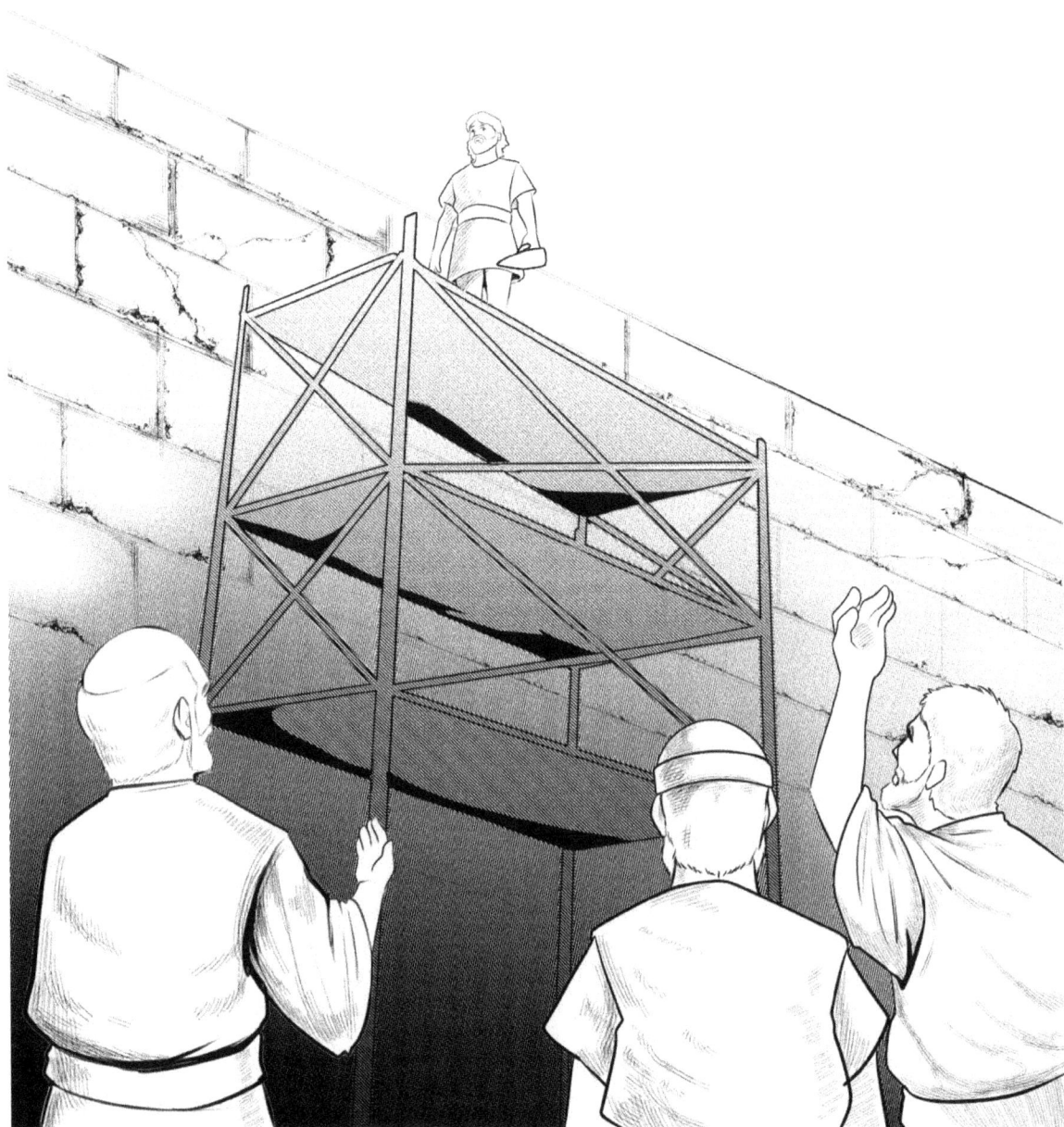

In record time, ahead of time, they finished the wall. It had only taken 52 days. Their unified community efforts enabled them to turn ruins into beauty.

The people and place were wholesome again, totally and fully restored. Past troubles became distant memories. This was a delight in Jerusalem – they had gone from ruins to restoration.

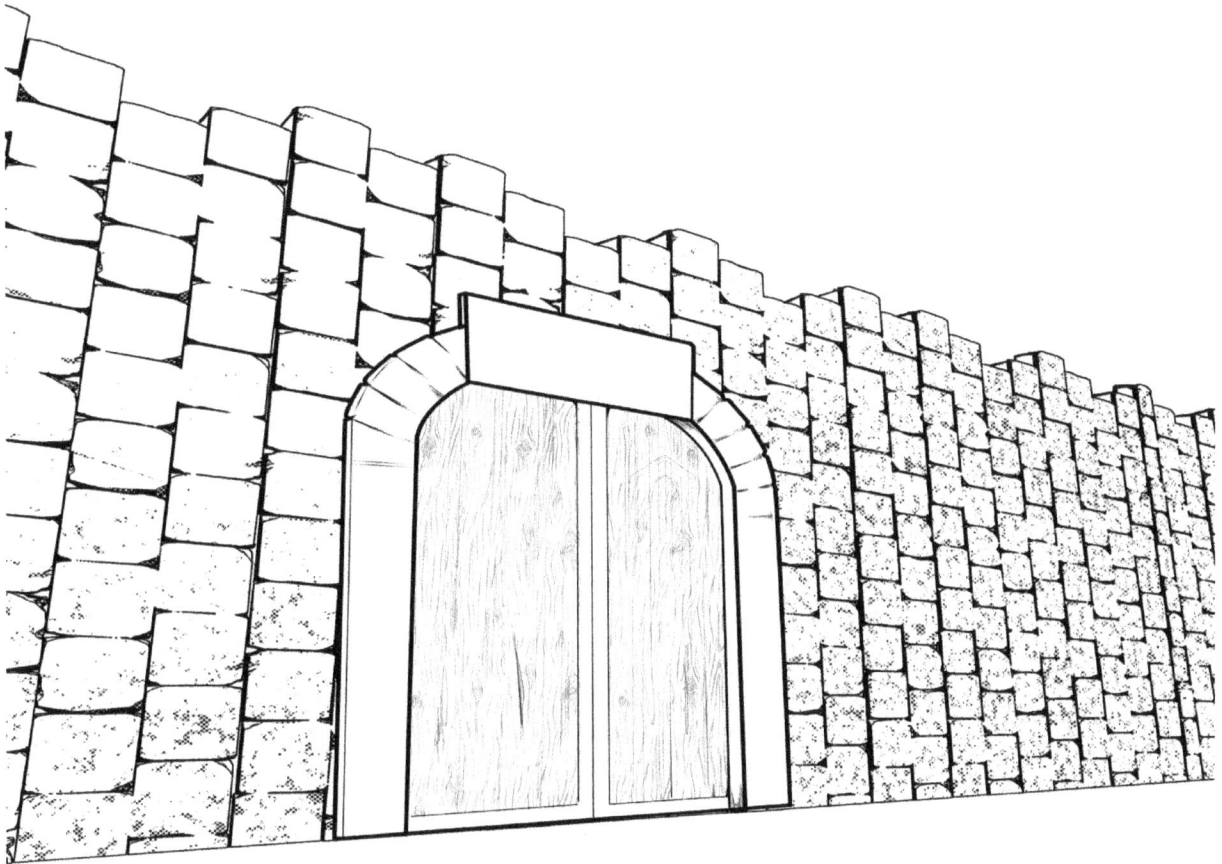

Gatekeepers, singers and set apart men were appointed by Nehemiah. Then Nehemiah called for a census, a registered count of people. Everyone had to return to their own towns for this.

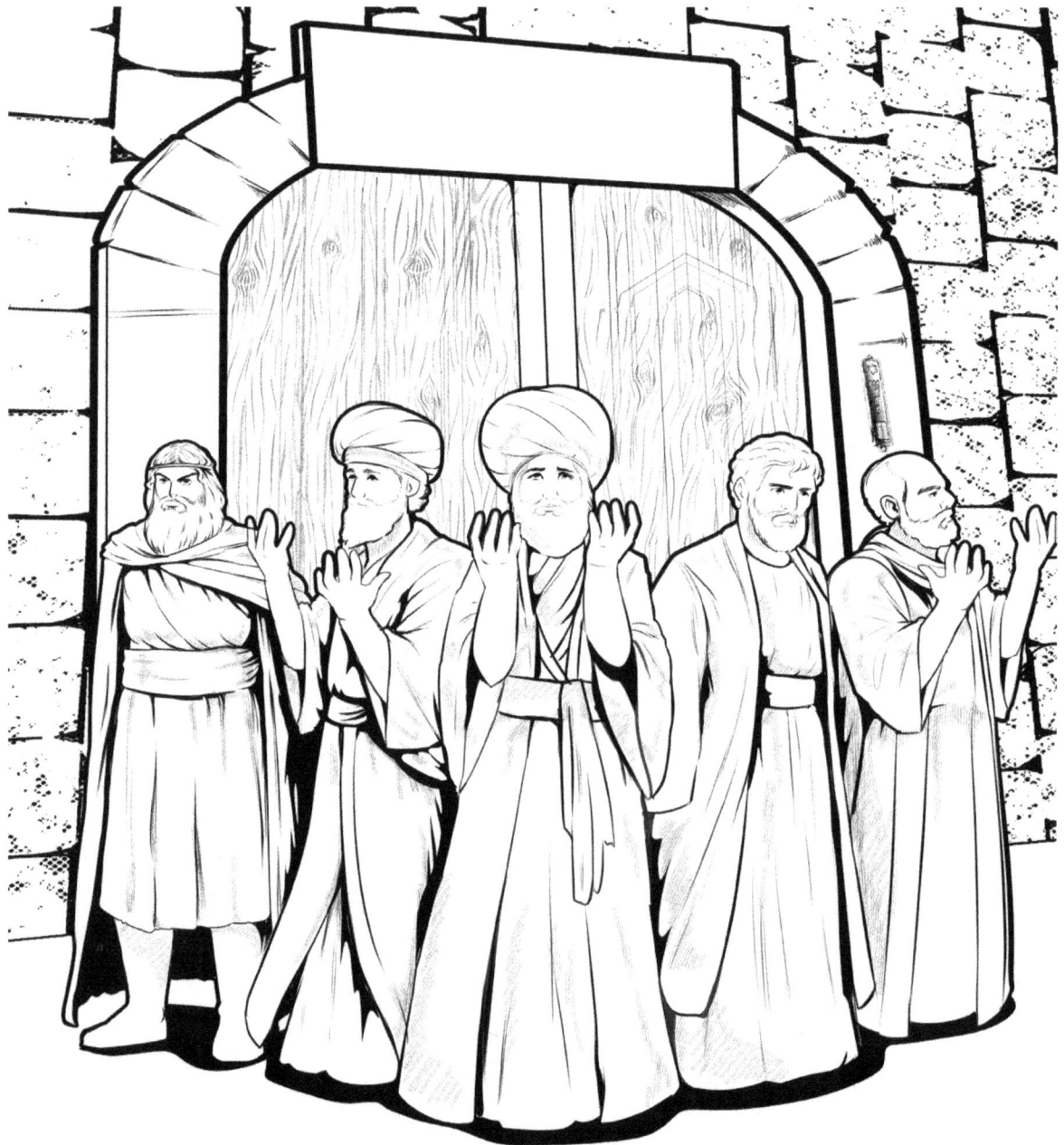

Ezra, the scribe, joined them. He led in the reading of the scriptures given by Moses, led them into a National Confession of Sin, had them take vows to follow God's law. He also helped get them back on track when they broke the vows.

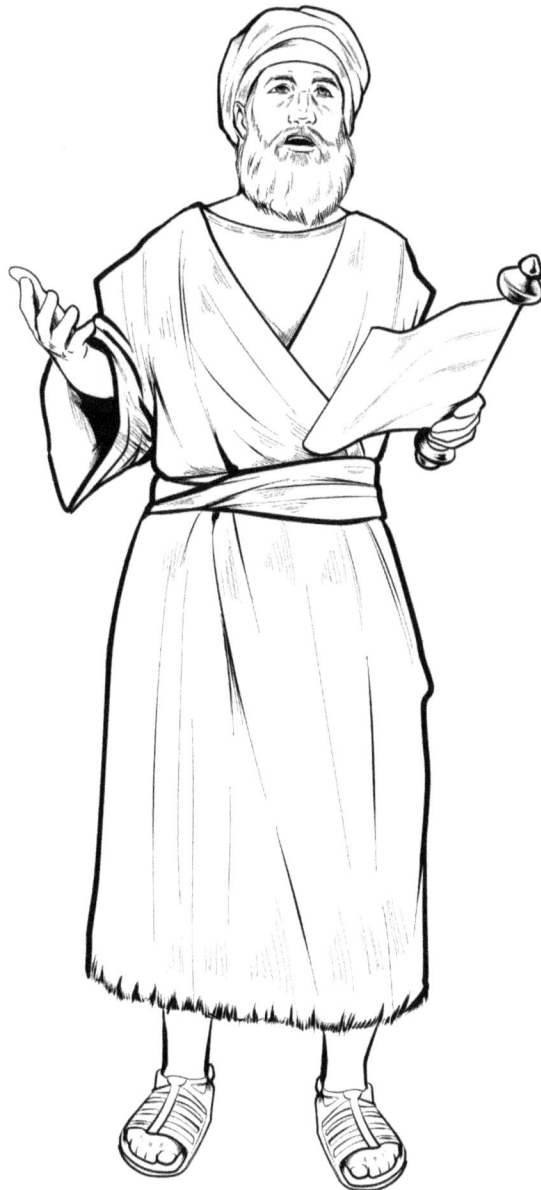

People began to go to Jerusalem and the towns around it to settle and live. They dedicated the wall that they had built. Walls were often wide enough for them to hold chariot races and high enough to fortify the city. Now human enemies, wild animals, bad weather and other threats were no longer a danger to those inside the walls.

It was a great celebration, with singers, a type of parade and the giving of thanks. Nehemiah prayed. "Remember me for this," he said to God Almighty as he named some things he had done to rebuild and reform in Jerusalem.

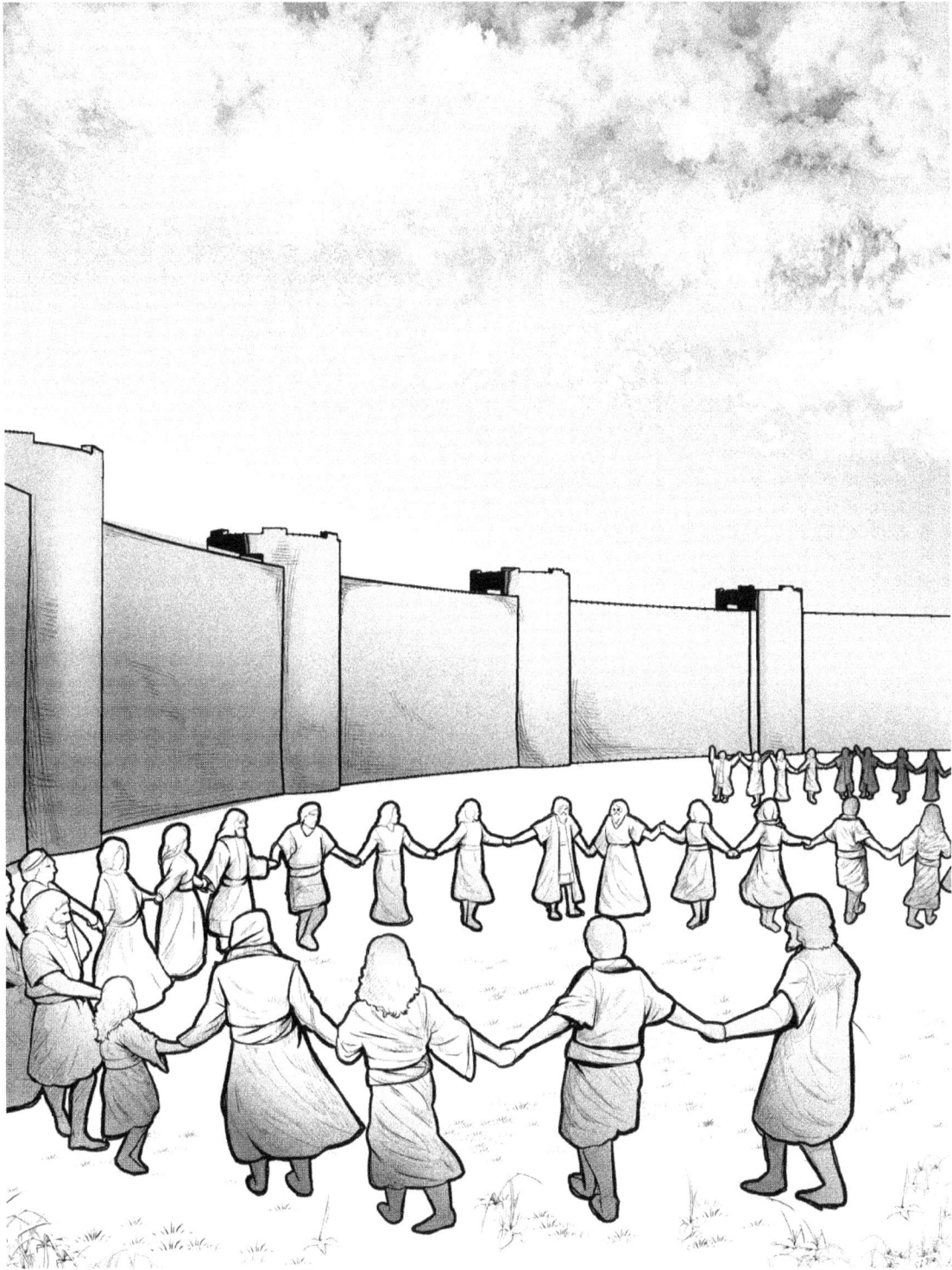

If you are not saved, are not 100% sure that if you died tonight that you would go to heaven, pray this Prayer to accept Jesus Christ into your heart:

I know I'm a sinner, and I ask for your forgiveness.
I believe Jesus Christ is Your Son. I believe that He died for my sin and that you raised Him to life.
I want to trust Him as my Savior and follow Him as Lord, from this day forward. Guide my life and help me to do your will.
I pray this in the name of Jesus. Amen."

If you have more questions, visit the link below or call 1-888-850-7479 and leave a voice message. Someone will call you back within 48 hours or less.

Billy Graham Evangelic Association
https://peacewithgod.net/

www.ingramcontent.com/pod-product-compliance
Lightning Source LLC
Chambersburg PA
CBHW040926050426
42334CB00061B/3475